Grandma's Ancient Beauty Remedies

From Her Kitchen Volume 6

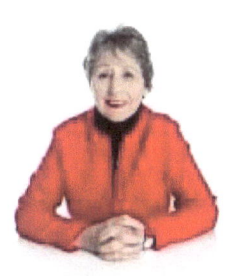 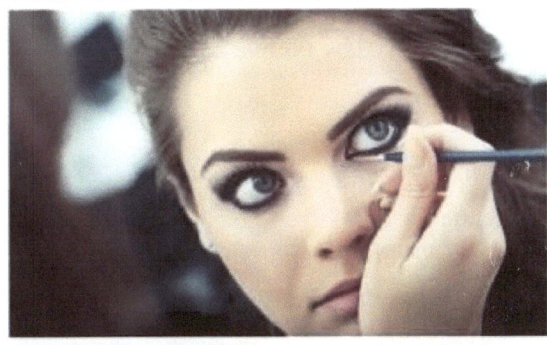

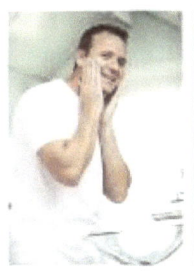 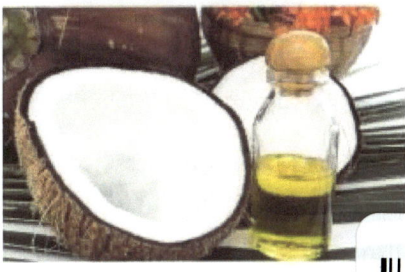 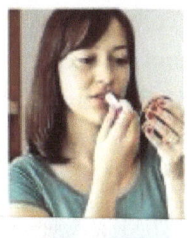

Dueep Jyot Singh

Natural Remedy Series

Mendon Cottage Books

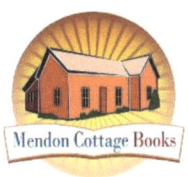

JD-Biz Publishing

Disclaimer

The information is this book is provided for informational purposes only. It is not intended to be used and medical advice or a substitute for proper medical treatment by a qualified health care provider. The information is believed to be accurate as presented based on research by the author.

The contents have not been evaluated by the U.S. Food and Drug Administration or any other Government or Health Organization and the contents in this book are not to be used to treat cure or prevent disease.

The author or publisher is not responsible for the use or safety of any diet, procedure or treatment mentioned in this book. The author or publisher is not responsible for errors or omissions that may exist.

Warning

The Book is for informational purposes only and before taking on any diet, treatment or medical procedure, it is recommended to consult with your primary health care provider.

Our books are available at

1. Amazon.com
2. Barnes and Noble
3. Itunes
4. Kobo
5. Smashwords
6. Google Play Books

Natural Kohl- eyeliner for your eyes

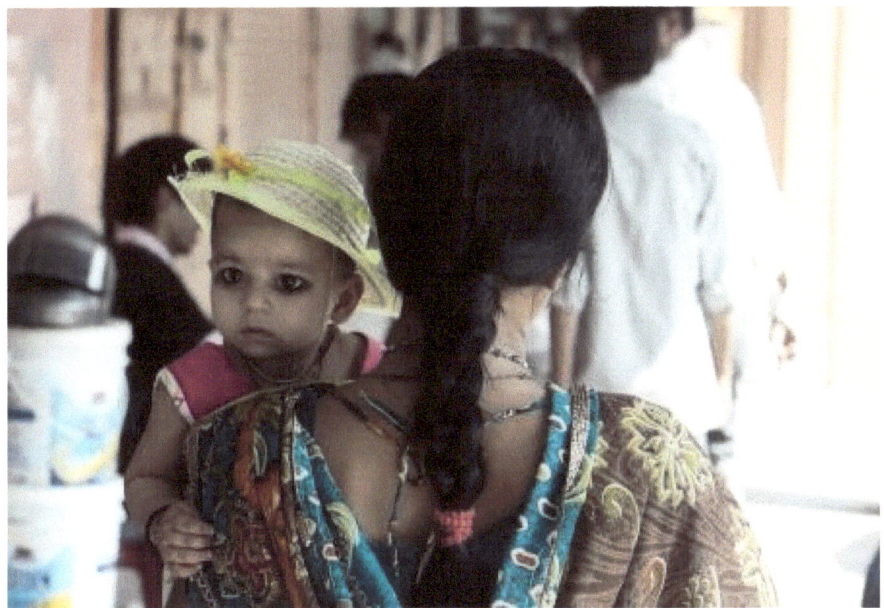

This little Indian baby has Kohl rimmed eyes , so that nobody can cast an evil eye on this beautiful little child, according to her mom!

This is the original ancient recipe, used by Egyptians and Indians to keep away the evil eye for millenniums. They never went out without outlining their eyes! The Egyptians, of course, did not use neem bark, because they did not know about it, but the Indians use it, to keep their eyes healthy and infection free.

Take a large lamp,- Diya (when I tried it, I used a small earthenware bowl.) Put some desi ghee, a handful of powdered almonds, a little bark of neem and a tiny piece of camphor in the lamp. Place it between two bricks. Light it. Now place a stainless steel cover upside down upon the bricks so that the soot can collect to be used as a natural heavy, healthy and dark application upon your eyes. Collect this soot and mix it with a couple of drops of ghee.

One of my friends in America says that it is very difficult to find pure Desi ghee and it is so expensive, so I am going to tell you the easy way of how to make this natural clarified butter at home.

She asked me whether it was okay she used castor oil, instead of this desi ghee. Castor oil stings, especially when you are applying it to your sensitive eye. If you are using this call as an eyeliner for your eyelids, then you can use Castor oil. But if you are using it to underlying the sensitive portions of your lower eye do not ever use Castor oil.

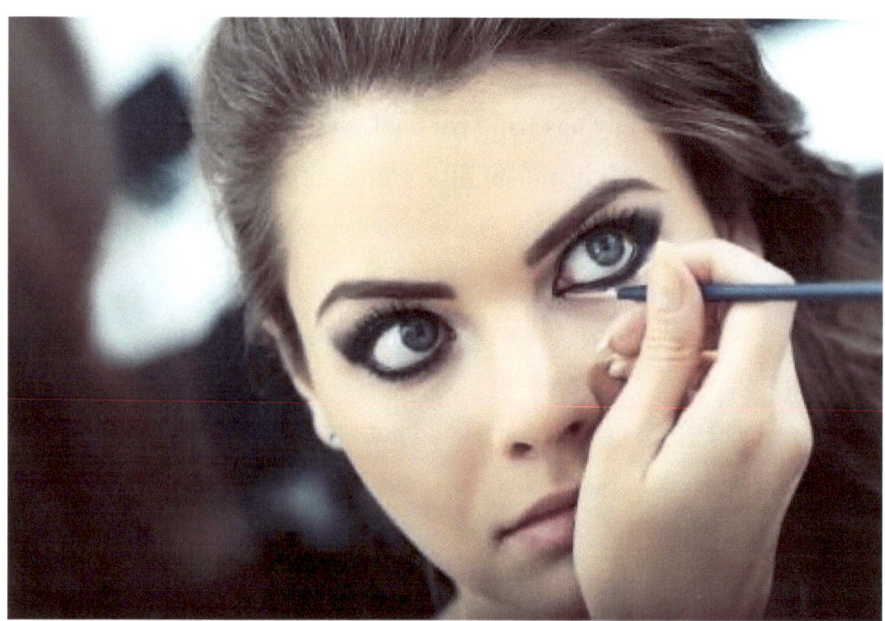

Do not use chemical-based eye makeup. Use natural Kohl.

Desi Ghee

Desi ghee is clarified butter, which is extremely concentrated and a very powerful healing agent. It is normally used in the making up of herbal medicines, because it is made of pure creamy milk butter. It is also used in making beauty creams, potions, lotions and other skin ointments.

It has a powerful aroma, and that is why only just a spoonful is added to fry meats. It is going to float on the surface of the meat dish, after it has been cooked, so you need to stir the gravy before serving. Also, the food is not going to taste greasy, even though it looks like it has been swimming in fat.

Desi ghee is the concentrated form of pure butter, which is heated to reduce the butter of all the impurities as well as moisture. This concentrated butter is normally used in Eastern cuisine, for searing meat, sautéing and frying food, because they offer its higher burning point. You make this at home by taking 2 pounds of best unsalted butter and melting it in a heavy bottomed pan. Allow the butter to liquefy on low heat for about 40 minutes. Maintain this simmering point, until all of the moisture in the butter has evaporated. The impurities are going to sink to the bottom of the pan. Remember to keep stirring the butter, so that it does not burn.

Pour off the clear butter and strain it through several thicknesses of muslin cloth. This butter is going to last for about a year, if it is placed in a cool and dry place. This butter is exorbitantly expensive. So in the East, people with easy access to plenty fresh milk make it right in their kitchens for crisp delicious frying results, and adding that taste of pure butter to all their dishes.

Skin Softener

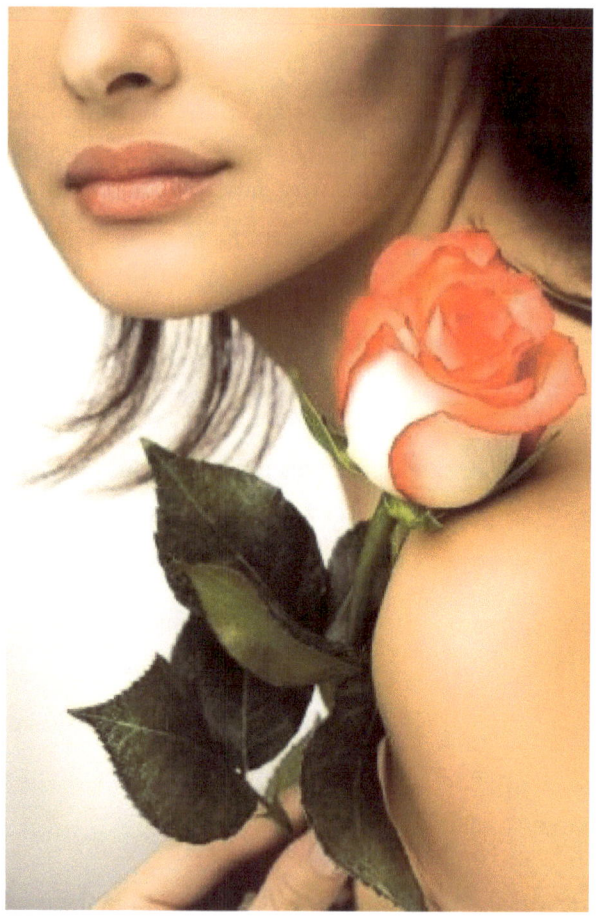

Mix the bread crumbs from two slices of bread and egg white of one egg. Put this mixture into vinegar, and allow it to stay in the shade for two days. Then bottle it and use it on your skin regularly to soften it.

Turmeric for Pimples and Spots

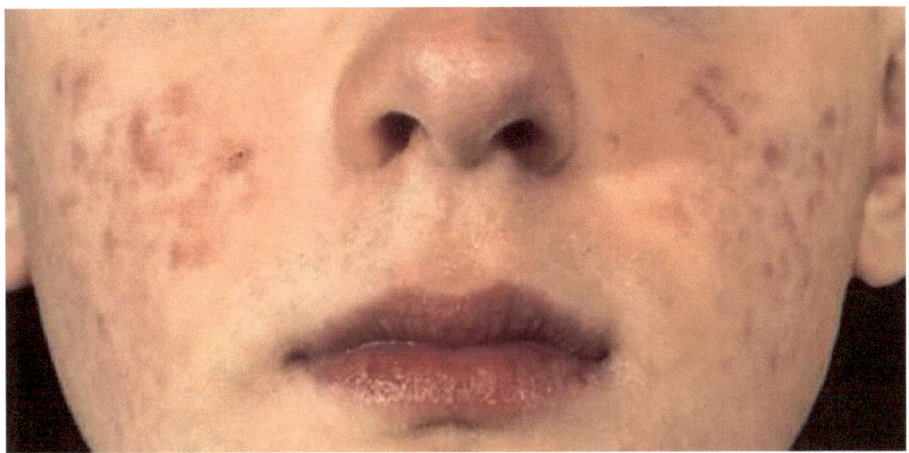

This is a natural remedy, which has been used for ages by grandmothers to prevent pimples and spots. Turmeric is also extremely useful in keeping your skin blemish free. Remember that turmeric stains, so if you find turmeric stains on your clothes, just apply some lemon juice on that affected area and put it out in the sun.

Roast some turmeric on the griddle, and powder it. You need a quarter teaspoon of roasted turmeric, 1 tablespoon full of honey and three pinches of salt. Dab this antiseptic cream on infected places, so that the honey can cure the infection and the turmeric can act as an antibiotic, as well as an anti-scarring agent.

The salt is for antiseptic purposes, and for keeping your skin bleached.

Turmeric Skin Cleanser

You may want to cleanse your skin with a mixture of milk cream, turmeric and salt, in the evening to keep it healthy, moisturized and glowing.

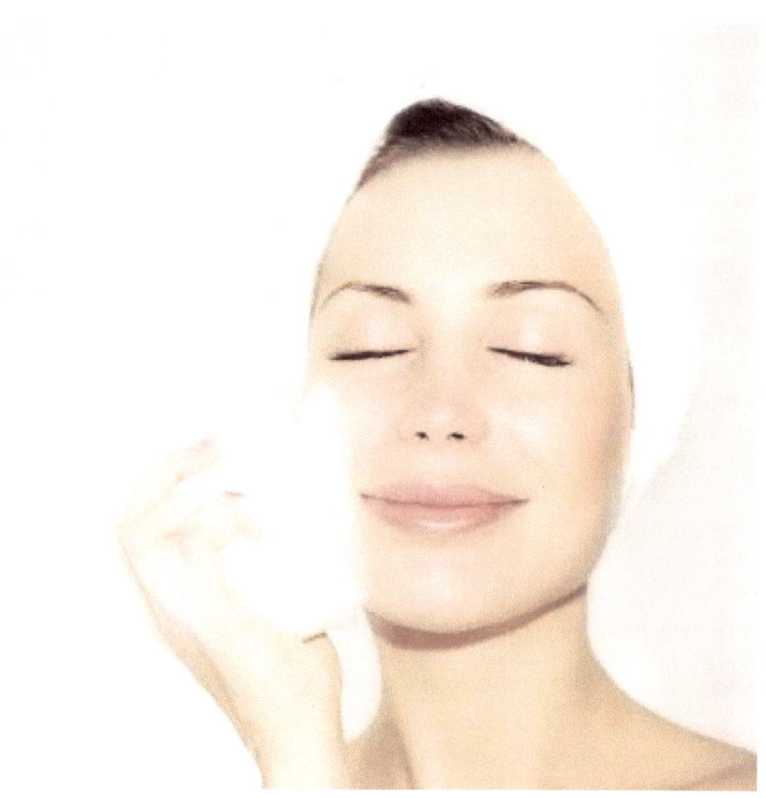

When you are applying a natural moisturizer around your mouth, do the applying in an upward motion – towards your forehead, and not towards your chin – this keeps the tissue around your mouth supple and youthful looking.

Turmeric Exfoliator

I am extremely fond of turmeric, especially in beauty remedies, and that is why I keep experimenting with it as an ingredient in natural beauty recipes. I normally used to use it in my facemasks, but I have also found that just a little bit of turmeric powder with cream rubbed all over my face and allow to dry is an extremely good exfoliator. And what about that golden yellow tint to my skin, brought about by turmeric? Well, just wash it off with soap and water!

Papaya Anti-wrinkle Facemask

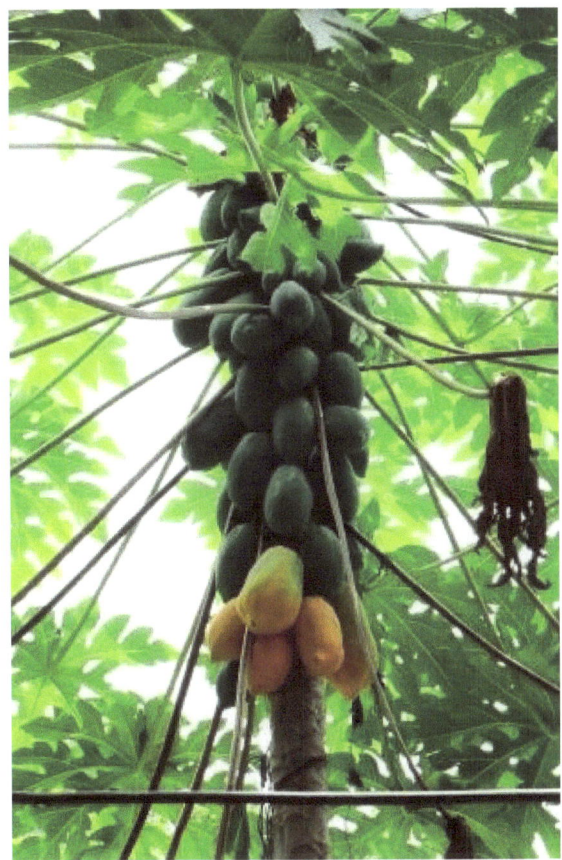

This recipe was given to me by a Thai friend, which is used regularly, in her family to keep the skin smooth, well, moisturized, glowing, well toned, and healthy.

Take out the pulp of one ripe Papaya, mix it with the juice of one lemon, and 1 tablespoon full of honey. Apply this paste all over your face and allow it to dry. Then rub off gently with warm water. This is the best anti-wrinkle facemask and should be done at least once a week.

Papayas are amazingly good antioxidants. But the pulp is powerful enough to encourage skin cell growth, so rubbing your face really hard to remove the dry pulp is going to make you look like a pink freshly plucked chicken.

Green Grape Juice

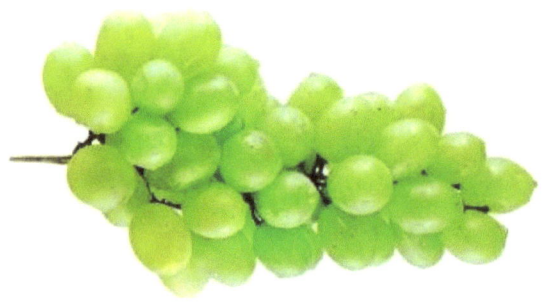

In the same way, applying the juice of mashed green grapes to the wrinkles and the fine lines and rinsing after 5 to 7 minutes, procedure repeated 2 to 3 times in a week is going to have wonderful results.

Almond Wrinkle Cure

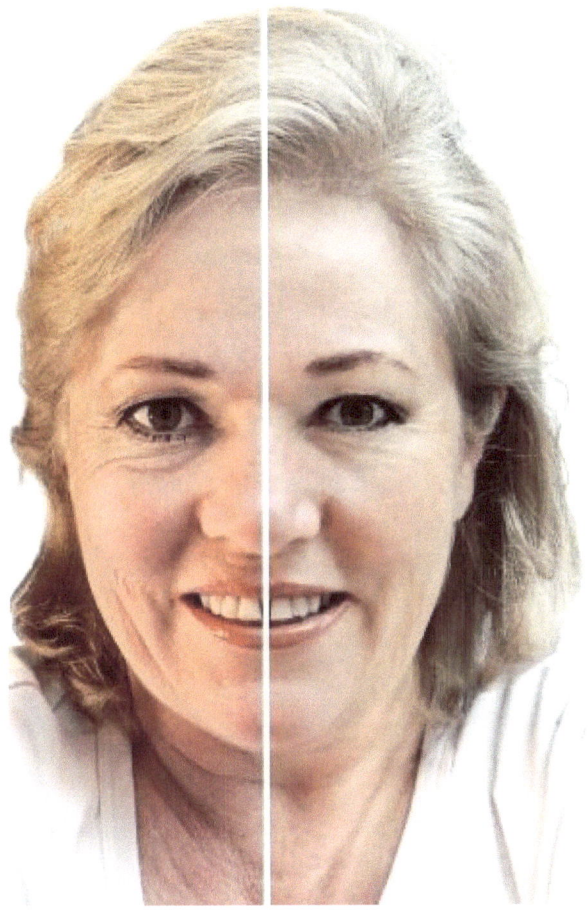

Get rid of wrinkles naturally

Now this is an ancient remedy, which was used by ladies in the East, to get rid of all the wrinkles. They soaked three almonds overnight in 3 tablespoons full of milk. Then the next morning, they ground up the almonds, possibly they drank up the milk, and/or applied it on their faces, with half a teaspoonful of honey. Leave this paste on for half an hour and then rinse with warm water or Rosewater, depending on your mood.

This was done regularly every day, and was an essential part of the beauty routine of those oriental lovelies who wanted to look ever youthful.

People reading grandma natural remedy books may find her repeating natural remedy cures, especially those of rose water. But that is because Rosewater is an essential ingredient of beauty in the East, since ancient times.

Who does not want to add the fragrance of the rose on her skin? This can easily be done by Rosewater. Queen Victoria perfume her gloves with rose essential oil, because that distracted her from the other smells permeating her vicinity, namely those of highly perfumed and unwashed bodies. However, as Rosewater is much easily made, and rose oil is so expensive, here is the way in which you can make rosewater right at home.

How To Make Rose Water

Rosewater is normally available in markets at exorbitant prices, but in India, anybody with access to the red rose - Rosa Damascena and a little bit of time enjoys making Rosewater at home. This Rosewater is used in cosmetics, as well as in cookery to impart the flavor of the Rose to your meal or to your skin.

Ingredients needed- 1 Cup Rose petals - 12 to 14 flowers.
2 cups water
Lots of ice.
A huge cooking pan - pan number one - with lid in which another pan - pan number two - can be placed comfortably.

Rosewater is just a matter of distillation. Put a wire stand in pan number one, on which you are going to stand the other pan number two. The condensed Rosewater is going to fall into pan number two.

Place the petals at the bottom of the pan number one. Now, cover the petals with water. Place pan number two on the wire stand. Now take the lid and place it upside down on pan number one, thus effectively covering the Rose petals, pan number two and the water. The Rose water is going to condense when you place the blocks and chunks of ice on the inverted lid.

You are going to have a cupful of precious distilled Rosewater, after 25 minutes of slow steaming of the Rose petals.

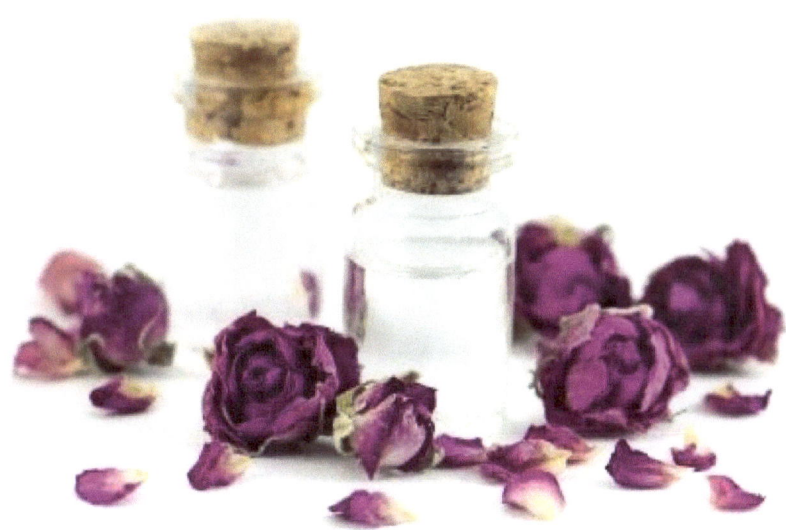

Precautions - Remember to have enough of water to cover the Rose petals. Also, it should not be of such a large quantity, that it displaces the wire stand.

This cooled water is now pure Rosewater. Pour it in a sterilized glass bottle. Use it to your heart's content. You may see a little bit of oil swimming over the surface of the water. This is Rose oil, and is even more precious. So if you used lots of petals in a larger pan, you may find even more Rose oil.

Reducing Age Spots

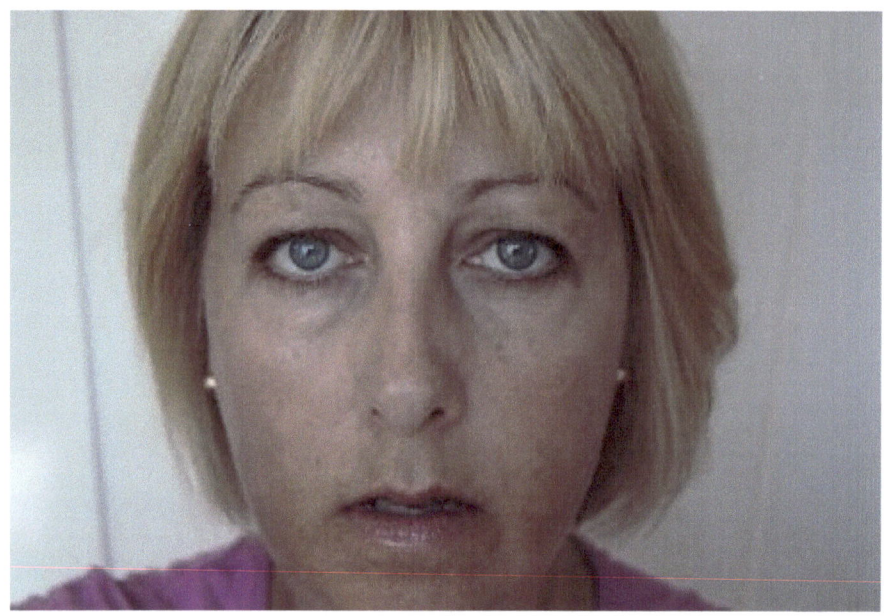

Too much sun damage can also cause age spots.

Take one part of onion juice and one part of apple cider vinegar. Apply this mixture with a cotton bud once a day to all the age spots, for at least six weeks. This is going to reduce them or make them fade away into the gloaming.

Removing Wrinkles and Fine Lines

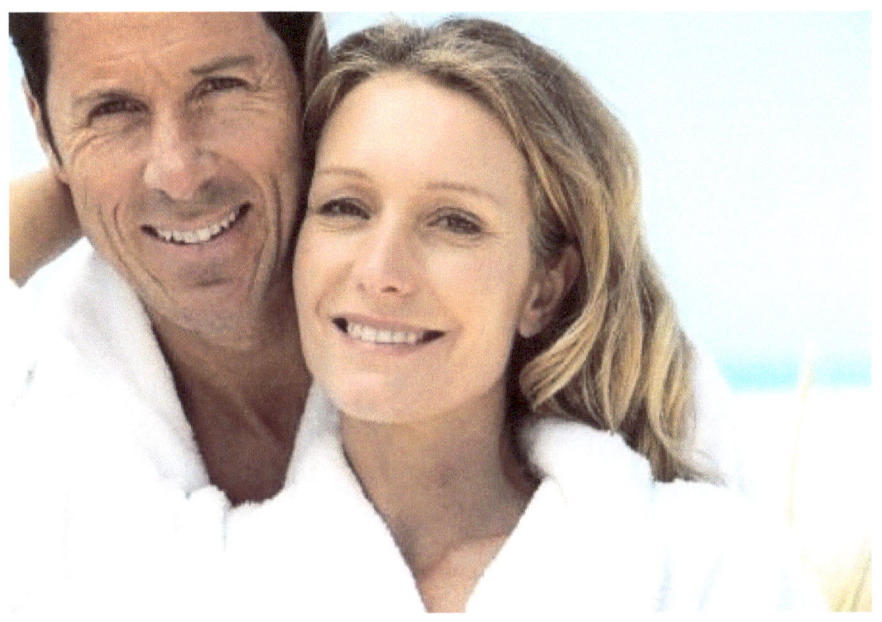

Wrinkles and fine lines can be reduced naturally.

Yogurt is delicious to eat. It is also an amazing way in which you can remove, fine lines and wrinkles. Take 3 tablespoons full of natural yogurt and add 1 tablespoon full of coconut oil to this mixture. Now slowly start applying it all over the fine lines and wrinkles. You may also use this as a facemask to moisturize your whole face. Allow the yogurt to dry on your skin. Now take a shower and moisturize again with coconut oil, after you come out of the shower.

Getting Rid of Dark Circles

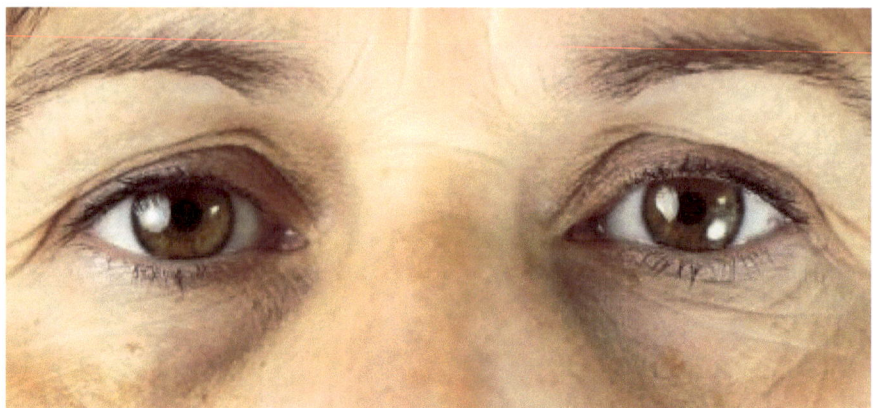

Dark circles normally happen when you are suffering sleepless nights. I am an occasional insomniac and that is why dark circles are part and parcel of my life. And that is why I am always on the lookout for natural remedies to get rid of these dark circles. The only way in which I can get rid of them is to go to sleep at 8 o'clock, and make sure my cell phone is switched off, until I wake up naturally, the next morning. Grandma would have made sure that I had plenty of spinach and iron in my diet, including liver , to encourage the red blood corpuscles growth. Because dark circles can also be caused due to anemia.

Take 15 to 20 mint leaves, and grind them with a little bit of water. Now apply this paste under your eyes and leave for half an hour before rinsing with warm water.

Here is another of my recipes to get rid of dark circles.

http://www.makeyourcosmetics.com/recipes/viewrec.asp?id=344&cat=facial

Different Types of Facemasks

Remember that all facemasks are not alike. Some nourish, some heal, some cleanse, some tone, some bleach .

Milk Facemask

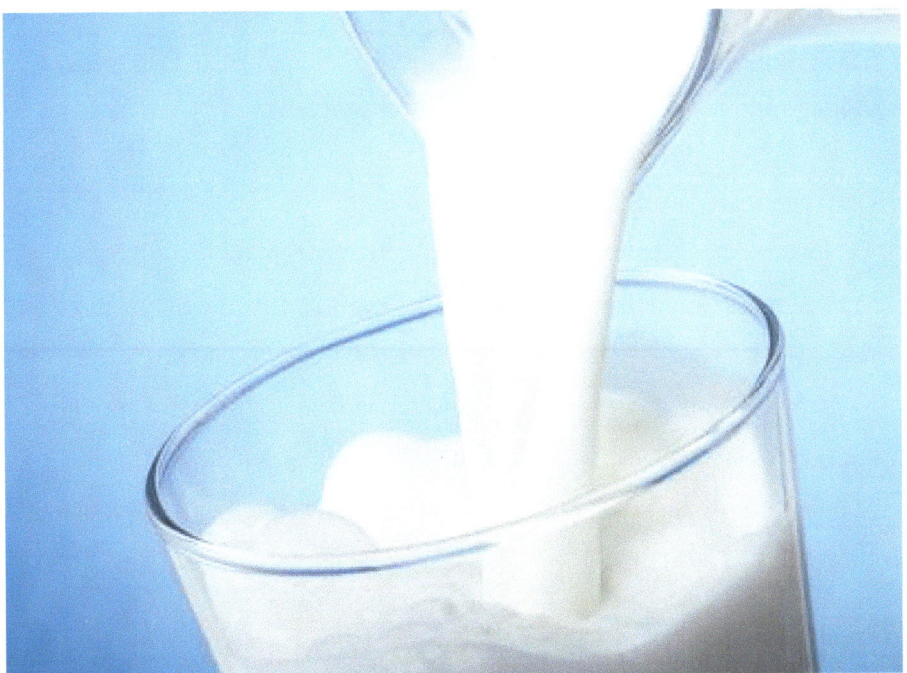

Just imagine not having anything in the home, to cleanse your face, except perhaps a drink of milk. Well, there you are, all you have to do is take a wad of cotton, dip it in milk and pat it all over your face. Let it remain on your

face for 30 minutes before washing it off with water. This is the best cleanser and nourisher.

Nourishing and Cleansing Mask – Carrot/Turnip

Boil a carrot and a turnip together. Make it into a paste. Keep this mask on your face for 15 minutes and then wash it off with milk.

Potatoes

You are going to use the mashed potatoes with Fullers earth. This is going to treat skin blemishes and get rid of all the dirt and grease. Add 3 tablespoons full of Fullers earth to an equal quantity of potato juice to make this mask. Rub off with warm water when dry.

Improve dull complexion

All you have to do is to mix 1 teaspoon each of cucumber juice, Rosewater, and lemon juice and apply it on your face. Keep on for 15 minutes and then wash. Well, That is suggested in the original recipe, but I do not bother to wash my face, afterwards. I like Rosewater, and lemon juice does not harm my skin. So no worries. You are going to see an improvement in your complexion within 3 to 4 days. Regular use of this remedy makes your skin glow.

Natural Skin Bleachers

There was a time when ladies used to use powdered lead outside of their faces, to show that they had a fair complexion. They also used to keep out of the sun, because having a suntanned skin was supposedly a mark of the working class, working in the sun and all Brown. Aristocrats, who stayed indoors, had an unhealthy sickly white/pale complexion, which was supposed to be very desirable. In fact, aristocratic ladies in the Middle Ages used to get themselves bleed it regularly, so that they looked all fragile and pale. And then, they died when still in their 20s because of loss of blood. The idea that you have to suffer in order to look beautiful is definitely not something that I advocate!

Fruit Juices

Lime juice, cucumber juice and carrot juice mixed in equal proportions and applied on your face for 15 minutes lightens your complexion. Detoxify your body, by drinking the rest of the juice.

Oatmeal Mask

Milk, oatmeal and lemon juice used as a mask is excellent for bleaching your complexion.

Sandalwood Facemask

Do you have sandalwood around you? A little bit of sandalwood powder, ground to a paste in milk and applied to your face, is considered to be an excellent facemask. In fact, natural facemasks sold by herbalists in India have this powder mixture, along with turmeric. So remember to add turmeric, while making up this facemask [1/4 teaspoon] and let it remain on for 15 – 20 minutes, before washing it off.

Anti-wrinkle Facemasks

Egg white, beaten well, spread on your face is going to iron out all the wrinkles, if left on for 15 minutes and then washed.

Barley, lemon juice and milk was used as a facemask by ancient Egyptians. You can also use it to get rid of the blemishes and keep your skin wrinkle free.

Beauty Lotions

Make your skin look great and feel good with lotions prepared from fruits and vegetables. In fact, Cleopatra supposedly had a bath with asses milk, but Queen Elizabeth the first kept her youthful looks for a long time by adding beer or wine foam to the bath water. She also made sure that she had some red wine added to the water, whenever she deigned to take a bath.

Diane de Poitiers was considered by many people to be a witch, especially by her Royal lover's legal wife, Catherine de Medici. She died at the age of 66, but looked extremely young and youthful until her dying day. That was because she ate a totally fruit and vegetable diet. Also, she was foolish enough to drink liquid gold, which she thought would keep her young, and that poisoned her ultimately instead of a de Medici poison.

Do not throw away the left over water, when you are cooking greens or boiling them. Spinach water is excellent to drink, and so is cabbage water.

You can also use them as face washing liquids, because they are rich in vitamins. These have to be used fresh.

Fairness Lotion

Take 3 teaspoons of cucumber juice. Add a pinch of turmeric and a few drops of lemon juice to this mixture. Apply and keep on your exposed hands, neck and face for half an hour. This is going to bleach your skin.

Pore Shrinking Lotion

Frozen tomatoes are of course the best way in which you can shrink pores. Put a tomato in the freezer. When it has completely frozen, take it out and mash it still in its frozen state. This is of course going to be done in the summer, when you can allow your skin to enjoy the feel of a cold, cold tomato pulp on it. Keep it on, till the frozen pulp reaches room temperature. Then allow the pulp to dry. This drastic action is going to close your pores. This takes about half an hour to occur. Now remove that tomato paste from your skin with cold water, and apply an ice cube over your tingling skin.

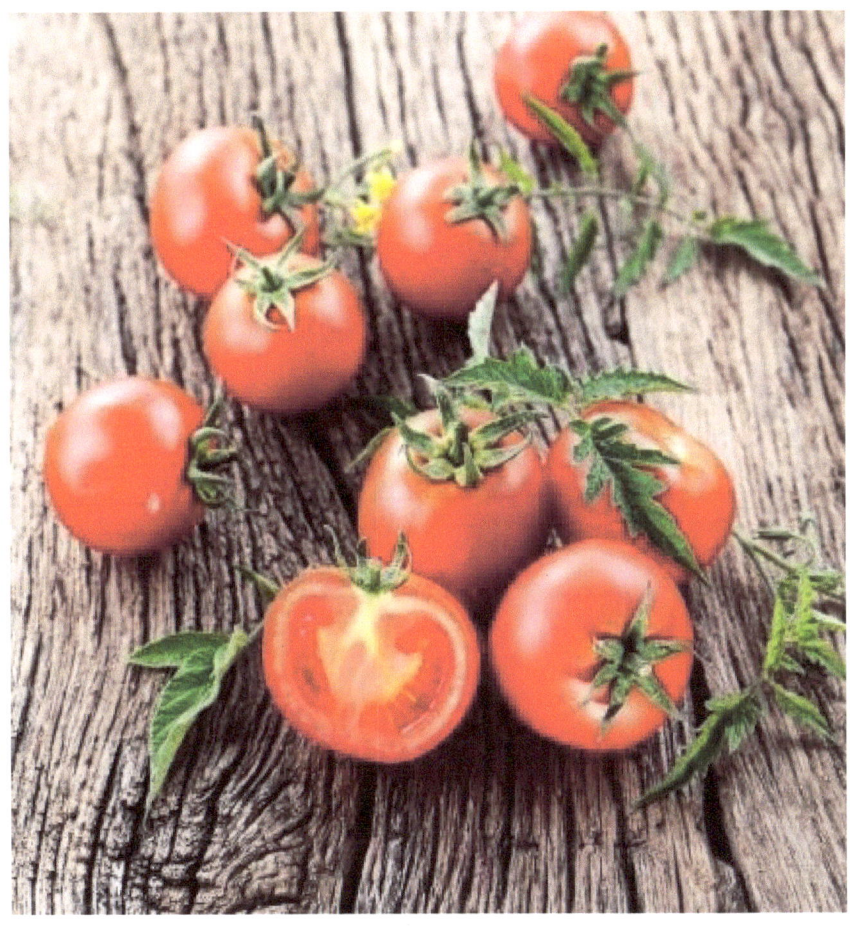

You can also use tomato juice with a few drops of lemon juice to shrink your pores, if you need this drastic treatment to be done within 15 minutes.

Bleaching Lotion for Sensitive Skins

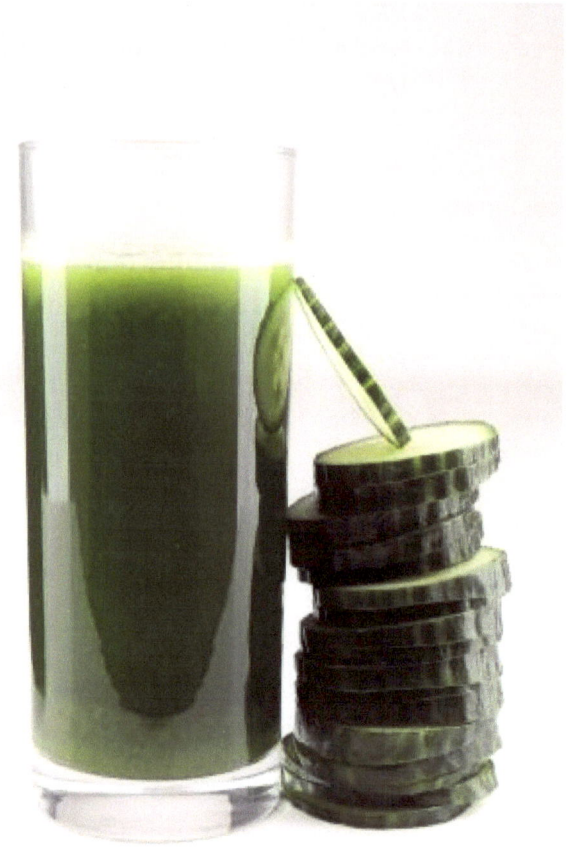

Take 3 teaspoons each of milk and cucumber juice, and add a few drops of rose water. Apply it on your neck and face. This is an excellent bleaching lotion, and you can either keep it on or wash off after 15 minutes.

Coconut Water Bleacher

Do you know that coconut water is an excellent bleacher? Just apply some coconut water, on your skin, when you are drinking fresh coconut water. By the time you finish eating the coconut meat and drink a polished juice, the coconut water is going to get absorbed in your skin. Wash your face. Feel it feeling soft and lighter in tone.

Cleansing Lotion

Take 2 tablespoons full of milk and cucumber juice. Add 15 drops of lemon juice to this mixture. Apply and then clean with a cotton wad after 15 minutes. When you add Rosewater to this mixture, it can become an excellent complexion tonic to make your skin glow.

Getting Rid of Sunburn

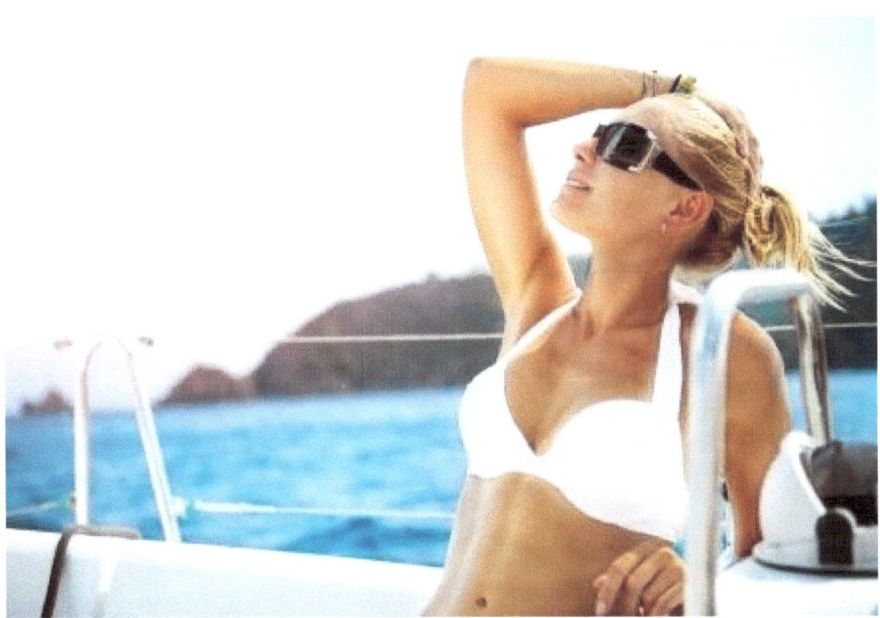

This remedy was used by women, we had to work on the farms in the sun. They took ¼ cup of buttermilk and added 2 teaspoons full of tomato juice. They left it on for half an hour before washing it off. They applied this on their skin and bleached it, thanks to the buttermilk. This gets rid of sunburn.

Greasy Skin

3 tablespoons full of apple juice, and 15 drops of lemon juice, make an excellent way to counteract greasy skin. Wash off after 20 minutes. Must be the malic acid in the apples, which gets rid of the grease and keeps your skin fresh smelling, and squeaky clean.

Tired Eyes

If grandma felt tired, she would go into her darkened bedroom, lie down with her feet raised a little, place these eye pads on her eyes, and just relax for a little while till somebody needed her.

These cotton pads were saturated in any of these following solutions to make effective refreshers for the eyes.

4 teaspoon each of lemon juice and iced water.

Ice cold juice of half a cucumber and rose water.

Cold black tea is of course Legion as a classic refresher for tired eyes.

Beauty Tips for Hair Care

Simple Hair Conditioner

Take an egg and beat it well. Add 4 teaspoons full each of honey and coconut oil. Mix well. This is a good conditioner. Massage well into your scalp.

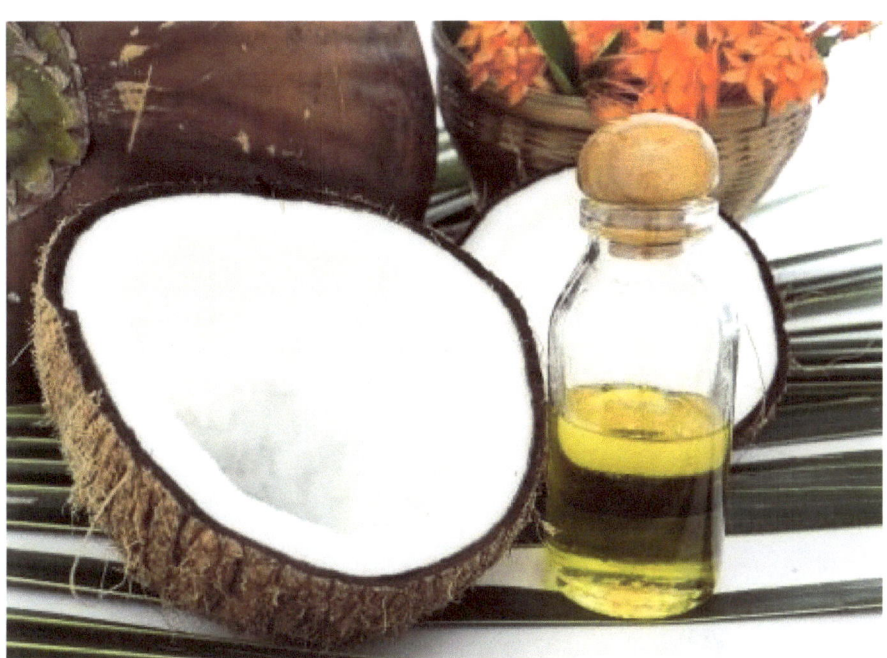

Place a towel over a utensil of hot water. Allow the steam to soak into the towel. Wrap your hair up in that towel for 20 minutes. This is going to allow the coconut oil to soak well into your scalp. Then shampoo with a shampoo made up of 125 g each of dried gooseberries, dried, powdered soap nuts and dried, powdered shikakai pods. This concoction has to be boiled for about 10 minutes, and cooled. Then strain it. You have a natural organic tonic shampoo, so throw away your chemical expensive hair damaging shampoos.

You can get all these powders ready and powdered in Indian grocery shops in the West, or you can get them online. Use this shampoo as if you are using your ordinary chemical-based shampoo. You are going to see a natural luster thanks to this milder shampoo, and due to the soap nuts. The Indian gooseberries, called amla have been used for centuries to promote hair growth and to keep them healthy, silky, and dark.

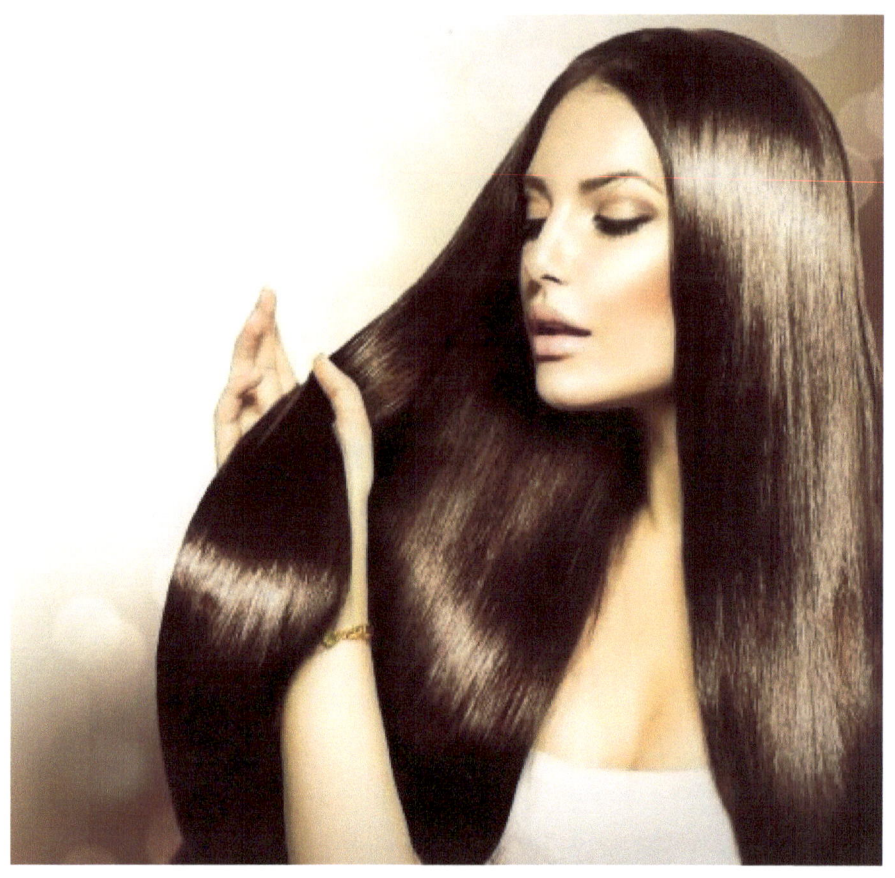

So if you want to try out this shampoo, just go to your friendly neighborhood natural products grocer and tell him you want amla-reetha-shikakai. All three of them go together and are pronounced aahm-laa-ree-thaa [or ray-tha]-shee kaa kayee said in one breath!

When you make tea and throw away the tea leaves, you are discarding a good hair care aide. Coffee grounds are excellent for giving your hair a reddish brown tint. Tea leaves darken your hair boiled. He left over tea leaves and use the water to wash your hair. It checks hair fall and makes your hair glossy and saw. Before the final rinse, add a dash of lemon juice to this water. It will give your hair a lustrous sheen.

Henna Shampoo

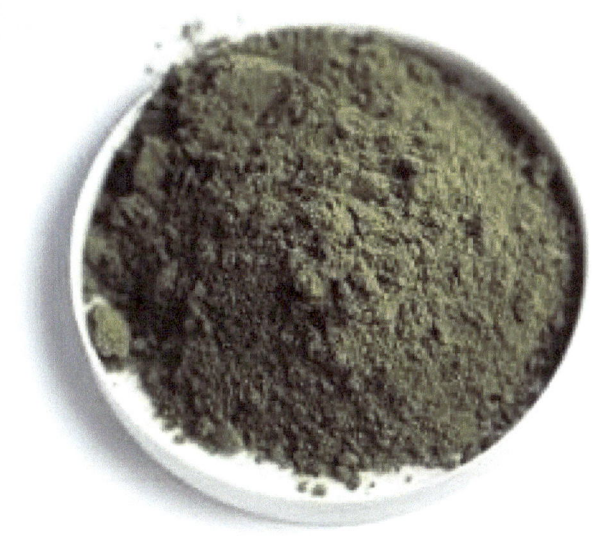

For all those people who want their hair auburn, Brown or reddish brown.

2 tablespoons henna

1 tablespoon sugar

2 tablespoons glycerin.

Half a teaspoonful filtered lime juice

6 tablespoons rosewater.

I am now using a chemical product, which even Victorian grandmothers used to make up shampoos. It is called **sodium lauryl ethyl sulfate – S LES**. You need 6 tablespoons full of this product. This gives you that foaming shampoo.

Mix and heat all the ingredients in a bowl over a hot water bath for five minutes. **Do not heat directly.** Take it off and let cool. Store in a glass bottle. You can add a few drops of your favorite perfume, if you wish. But I think rosewater is enough, is not it.

Hair Cream

3 tablespoons petroleum jelly.(Stop Press – Vaseline is the brand-name for hundred percent petroleum jelly with a little bit of perfume added to it!]

3 tablespoons castor oil.
3 tablespoons coconut hair oil, or any other natural or herbal hair oil.
3 tablespoons emulsifying wax
Heat all the ingredients over a water bath, until they have been melted properly. Mix well, and add a little bit of perfume if you want your hair cream, smelling of roses, or jasmine or bay rum for men!

Bay Rum after Shave Lotion for Men

This is something extremely unusual, which I came across, about how bay rum was made. This is what is normally used in aftershave lotions. But the original recipe was found by a 16th-century sailor, who found himself in Jamaica and noticed that just rubbing bay leaves all over his body left it smelling nice and macho.

So here is the recipe for Bay rum aftershave lotion for men.

As the recipe suggests, it is going to be a mixture of Bay leaves and Jamaican rum.

Do not buy the cooking bay leaf available at your nearest grocery store. Instead, ask for dried Pimenta racemosa leaves. This is the original Jamaican bay leaf, which is used to make the aftershave. You can get them at natural product shops and organic food stores.

2 tablespoons heaped of Jamaica rum

115 g Vodka-roughly 4 ounces

You can use your own spices like cinnamon, Rosemary, allspice, lavender, Juniper or any other nice smelling spices, to add the spicy smell to this aftershave. Also add the zest of one orange.

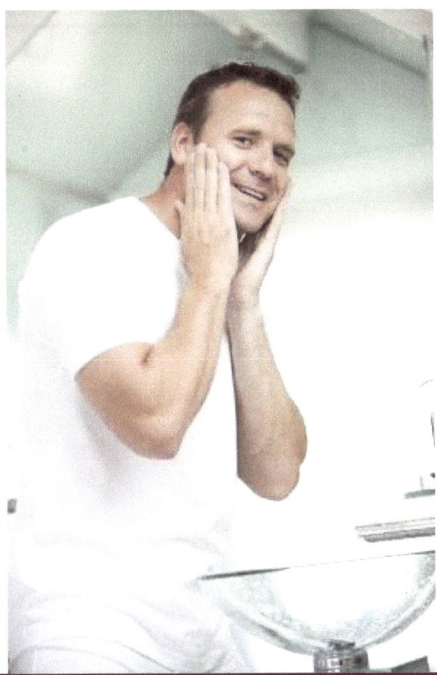

Mix all these contents together, in one glass jar. Put this into your cellar, in a cool dark place for about two weeks. That means the essential oils are going to be incorporated in the alcohol. After that, strain the end product, and continue repeating till there is absolutely no residue left in the liquid. Put in a glass bottle of your choice, and use after shaving as a splash.

I guess this was the masculine scent so favored by Victorian and Edwardian writers, when they talked about their macho Dell and Glyn type alpha heroes, coming into the room with the smell of horse and bay rum, following them. This scent would have been virile and overpowering enough to have all their languishing and overtly sentimental heroines swooning away daintily at those well shod – in – riding – boots- feet.

Corn Flour Hand Cream

This can be made with 1/8 cups each of glycerin and flour and 1 cup of water. Heat the glycerin and water in a pan on medium flame. Add the flour slowly until the mixture thickens. Take it off the heat, when the mixture has reached a cream like consistency.

Cool. Add the juice of one lemon, and some rosewater to this mixture and put it in a bottle. Use on your hands, whenever they want some pampering – that means every evening.

Well, do not say that grandma did not have what is now called a beauty parlor, right in her kitchen. Grandpa at that time may not have worried over much over powders, paints and lotions, but he also knew how to keep himself sweet smelling with fragrances and essences. Grandpa also used a mixture of wax and suet with fragrances on his hair, to keep it well styled and in place. Fact, the ancient Greeks and Romans anointed themselves with these sweet smelling fragrant oils three times a day, so that the smell never quite went away!

Ancient Lip Salve

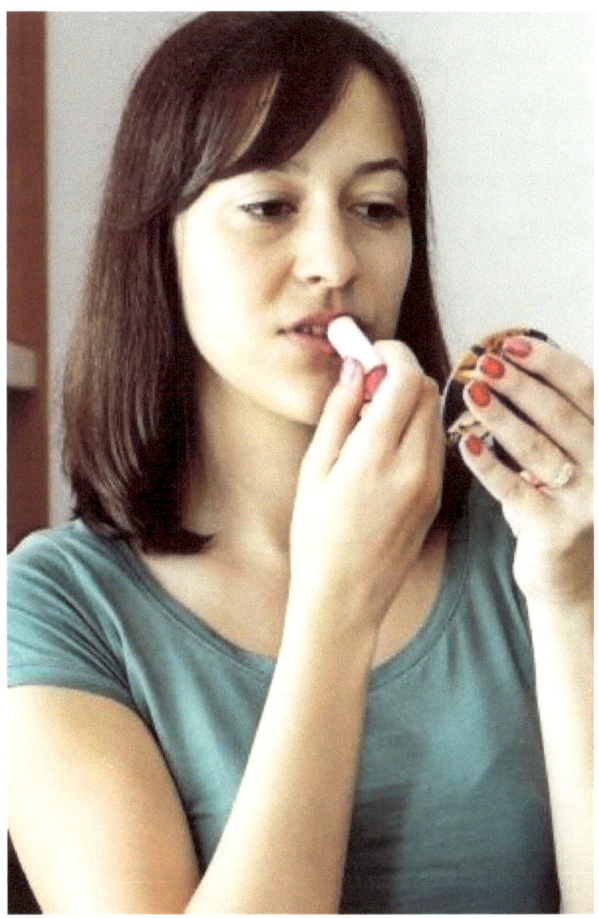

Here is an amusing way in which you can make a lip salve, taken from an ancient recipe book. I am giving you the modern English description without ye olde wordes confusing the reader interested in lip salves or what we call now lipsticks.

Take equal parts of lard and suet. Add some alkanet root to it. Every pound of Salve should have an ounce of bergamot added to it. Now place this in the vessel and melt all these together over a hot bath. Once it has been poured into the container and is cool, heat a red hot iron and hold above the container's mouth, so that the surface of the salve is melted and is smooth.

Well, my 21st century suggestion is use lanolin, wax and spermaceti. Put in some powdered alkanet and bergamot. Pour in lipstick mold and you have natural lipstick.

Conclusion

Now that you know all about the power of ancient natural remedies, is it surprising that these recipes are being "discovered" by beauty product manufacturing brand names and are being sold to you in expensively backed bottles.

Natural beauty products are getting to be more in vogue, nowadays, because you and other ladies are starting to understand how dangerous some of the things we have been putting next to our skin can be.

Author Bio

Dueep Jyot Singh is a Management and IT Professional who managed to gather Postgraduate qualifications in Management and English and Degrees in Science, French and Education while pursuing different enjoyable career options like being an hospital administrator, IT,SEO and HRD Database Manager/ trainer, movie scriptwriter, theatre artiste and public speaker, lecturer in French, Marketing and Advertising, ex-Editor of Hearts On Fire (now known as Solsctice) Books Missouri USA, advice columnist and cartoonist, publisher and Aviation School trainer, ex- moderator on Medico.in, banker, student councilor ,travelogue writer … among other things! One fine morning, she decided that she had enough of killing herself by Degrees and went back to her first love -- writing. It's more enjoyable! She already has 48 published academic and 14 fiction- in- different- genre books under her belt.

When she is not designing websites or making Graphic design illustrations for clients , she is browsing through old bookshops hunting for treasures, of which she has an enviable collection – including R.L. Stevenson, O.Henry, Dornford Yates, Maurice Walsh, C.N.Williamson, Sapper, Bartimeus and the crown of her collection- Dickens "The Old Curiosity Shop," and so on… Just call her "Renaissance Woman" - collecting herbal remedies, acting like Universal Helping Hand/Agony Aunt, or escaping to her dear mountains for a bit of exploring, collecting herbs and plants, and trekking.

Check out some of the other JD-Biz Publishing books

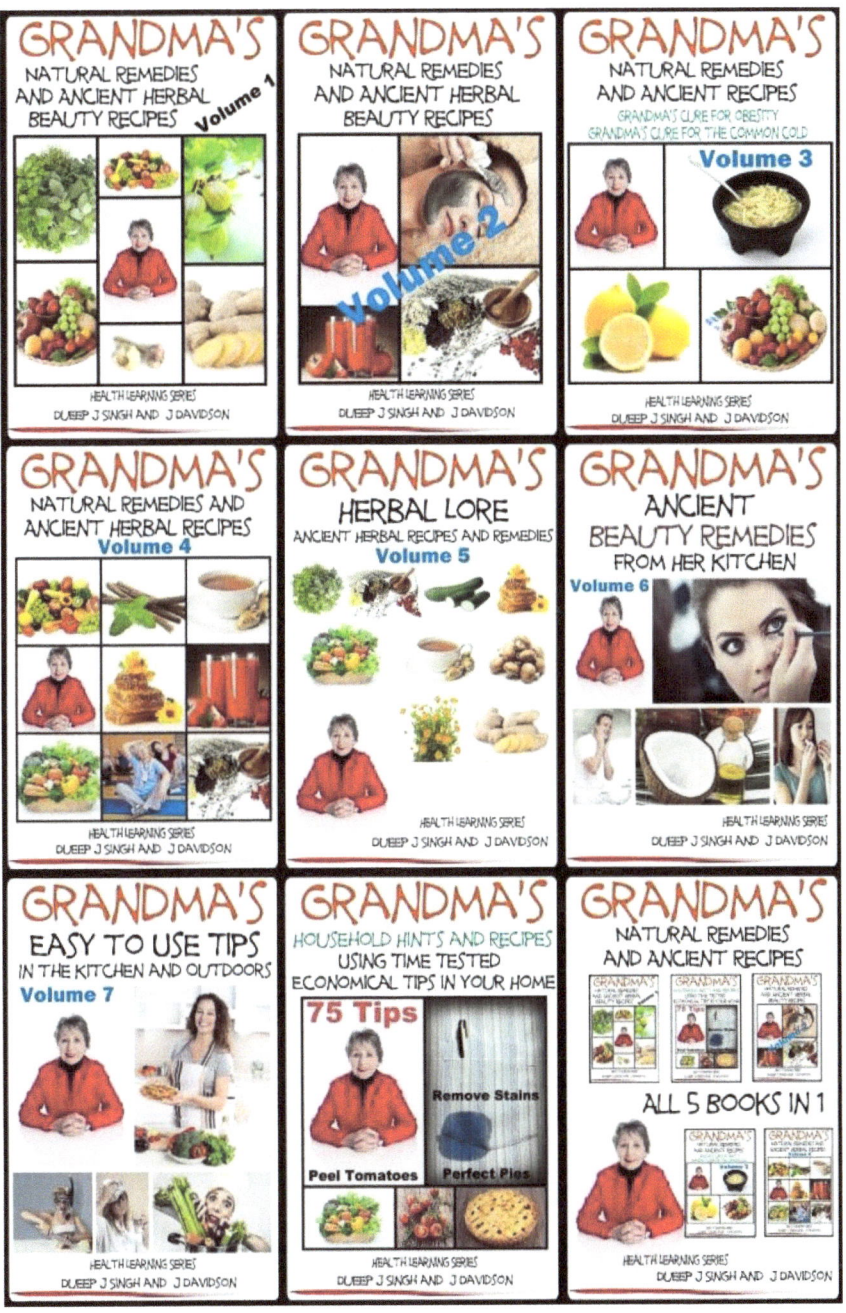

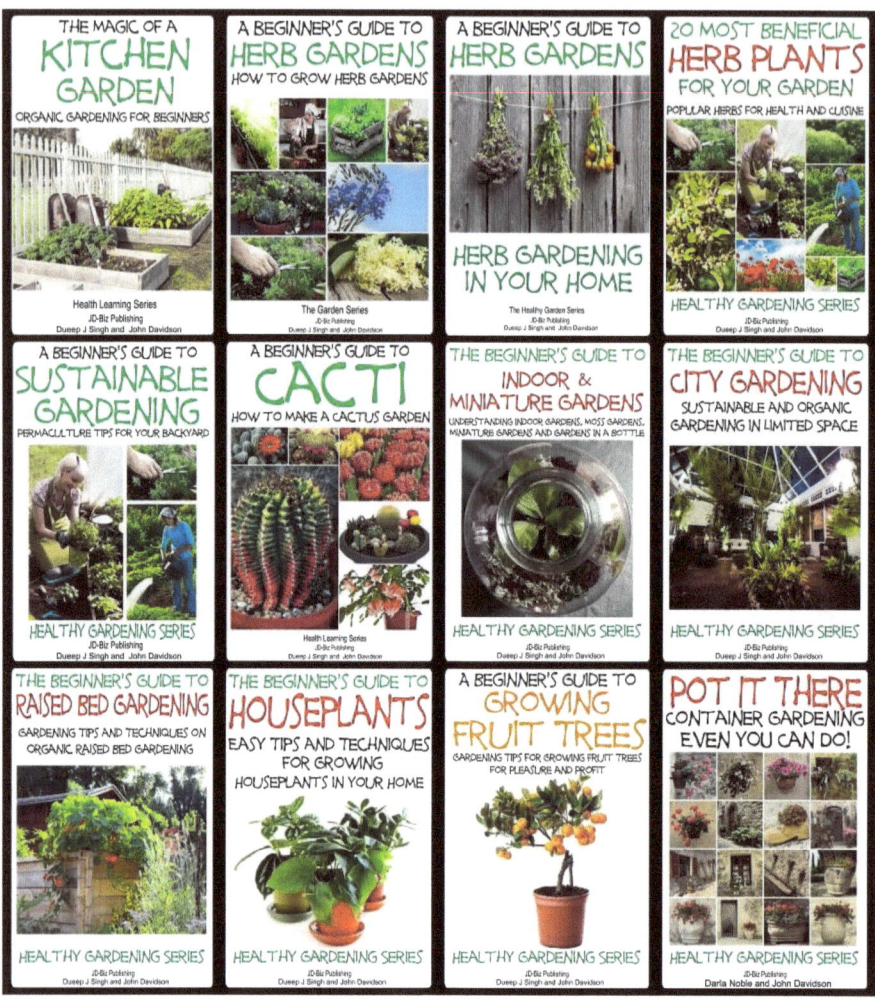

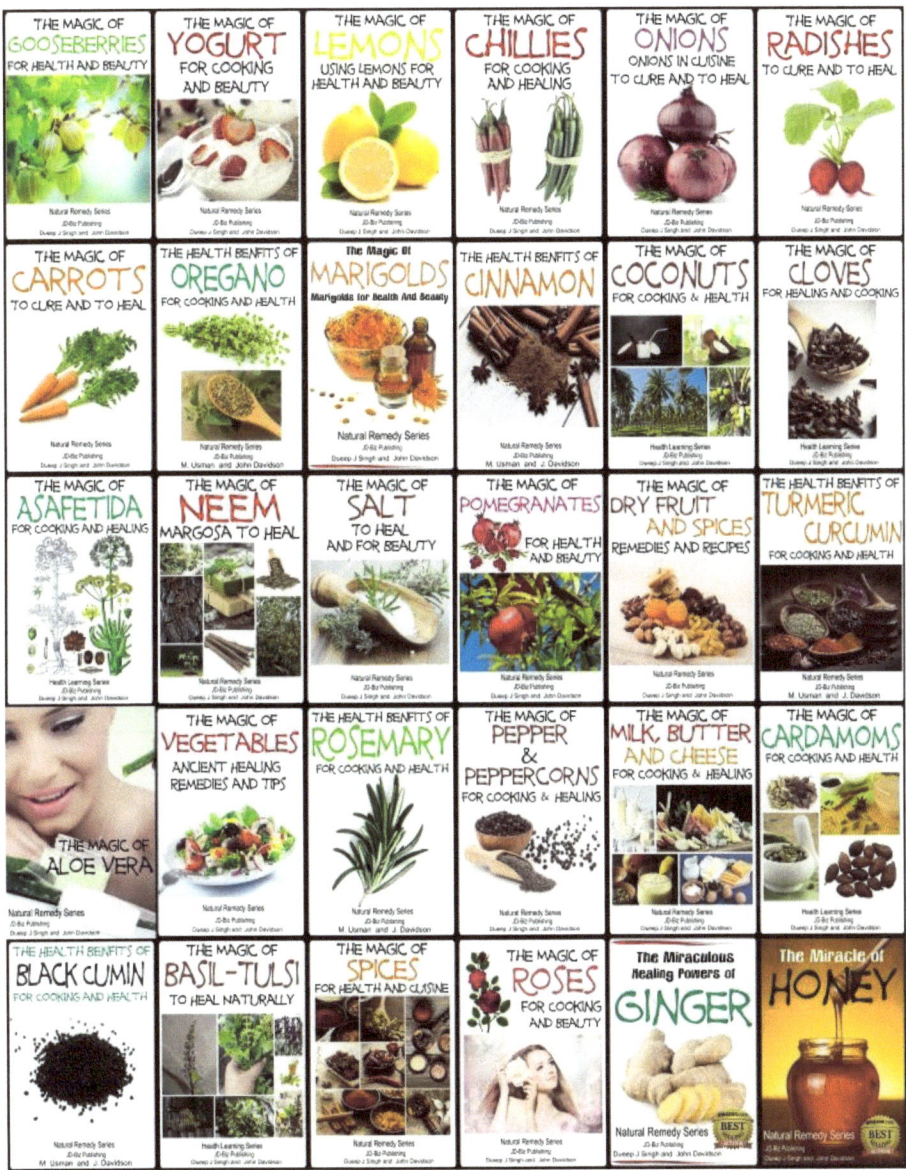

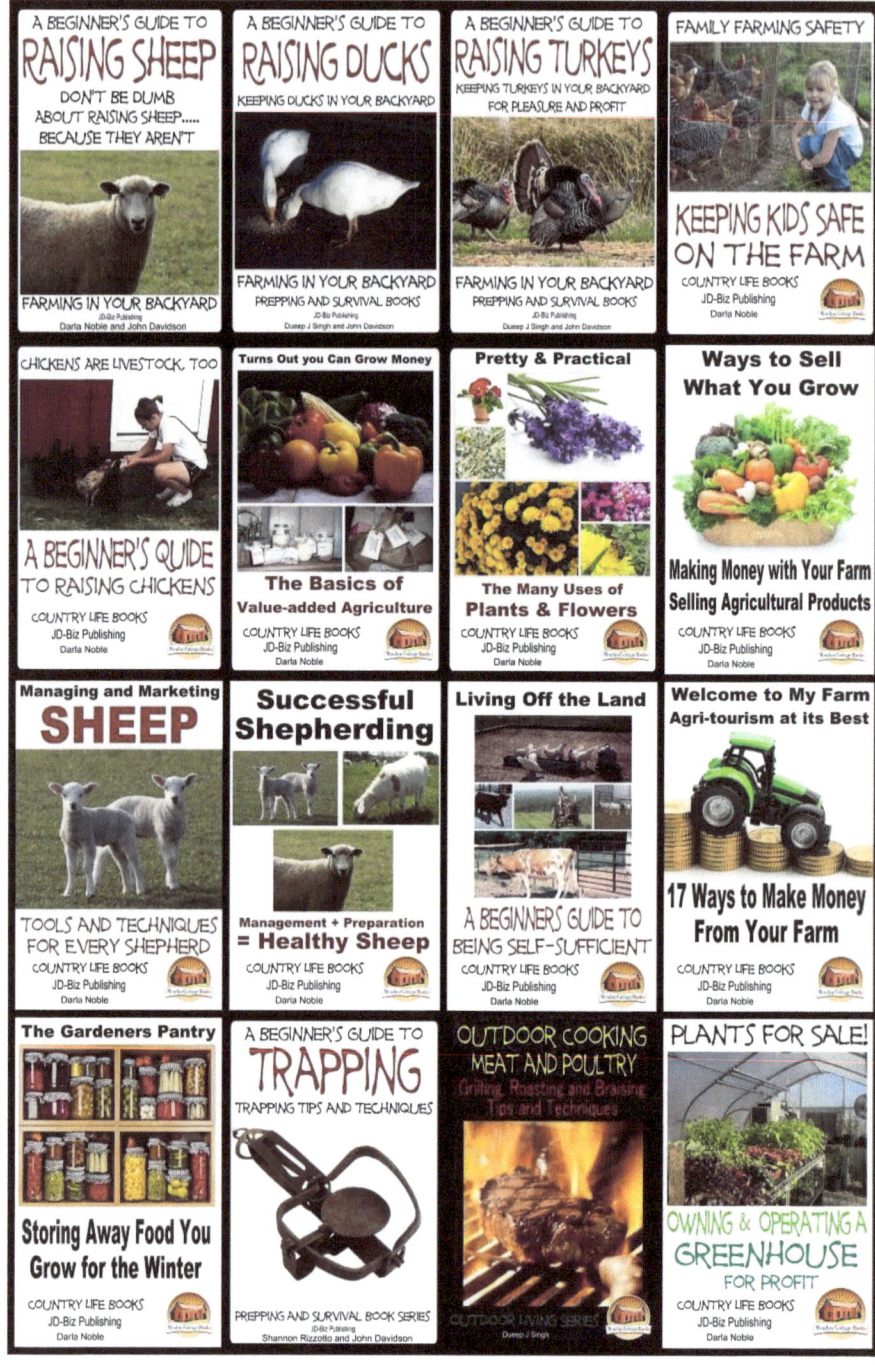

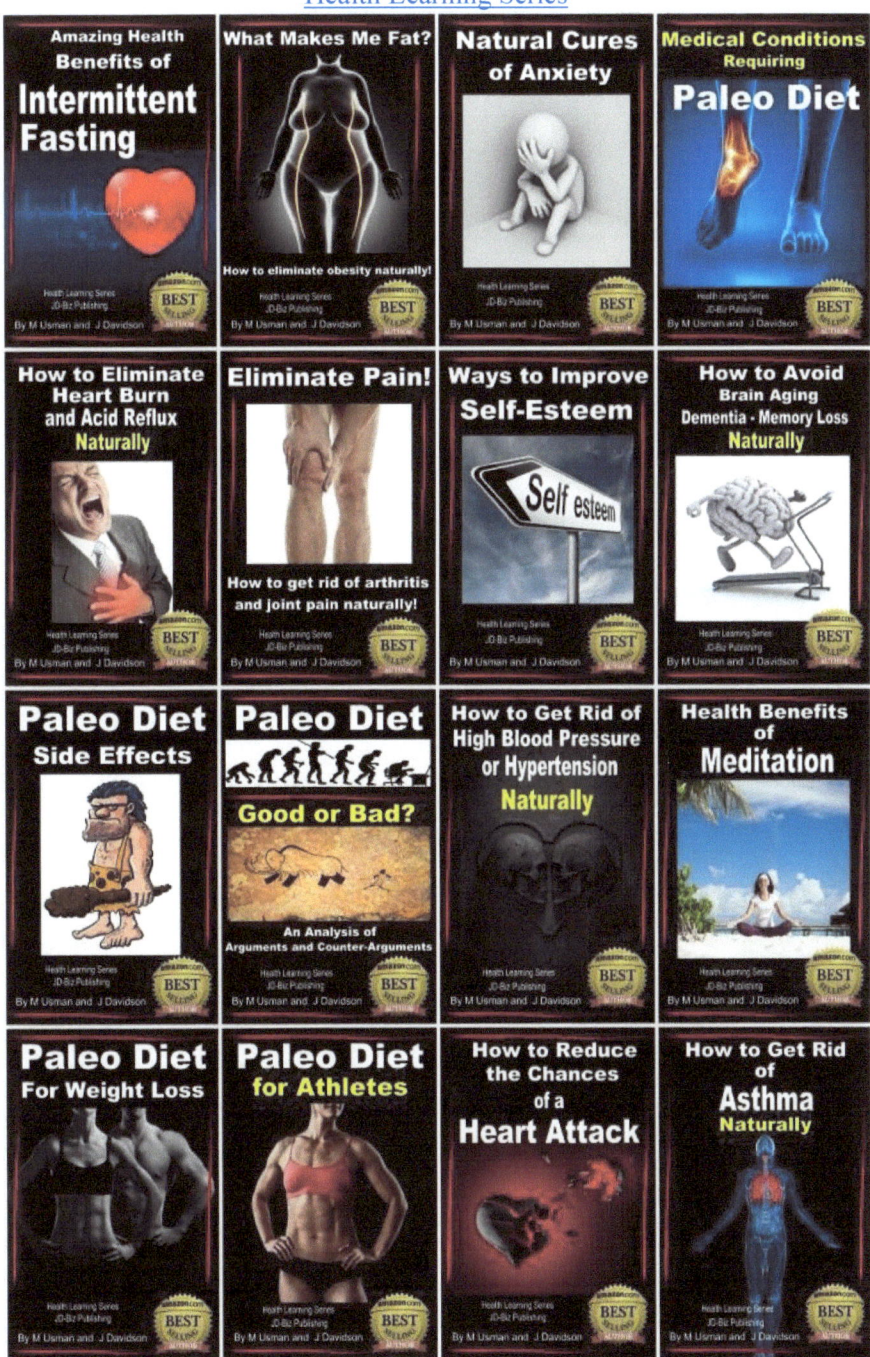

Amazing Animal Book Series

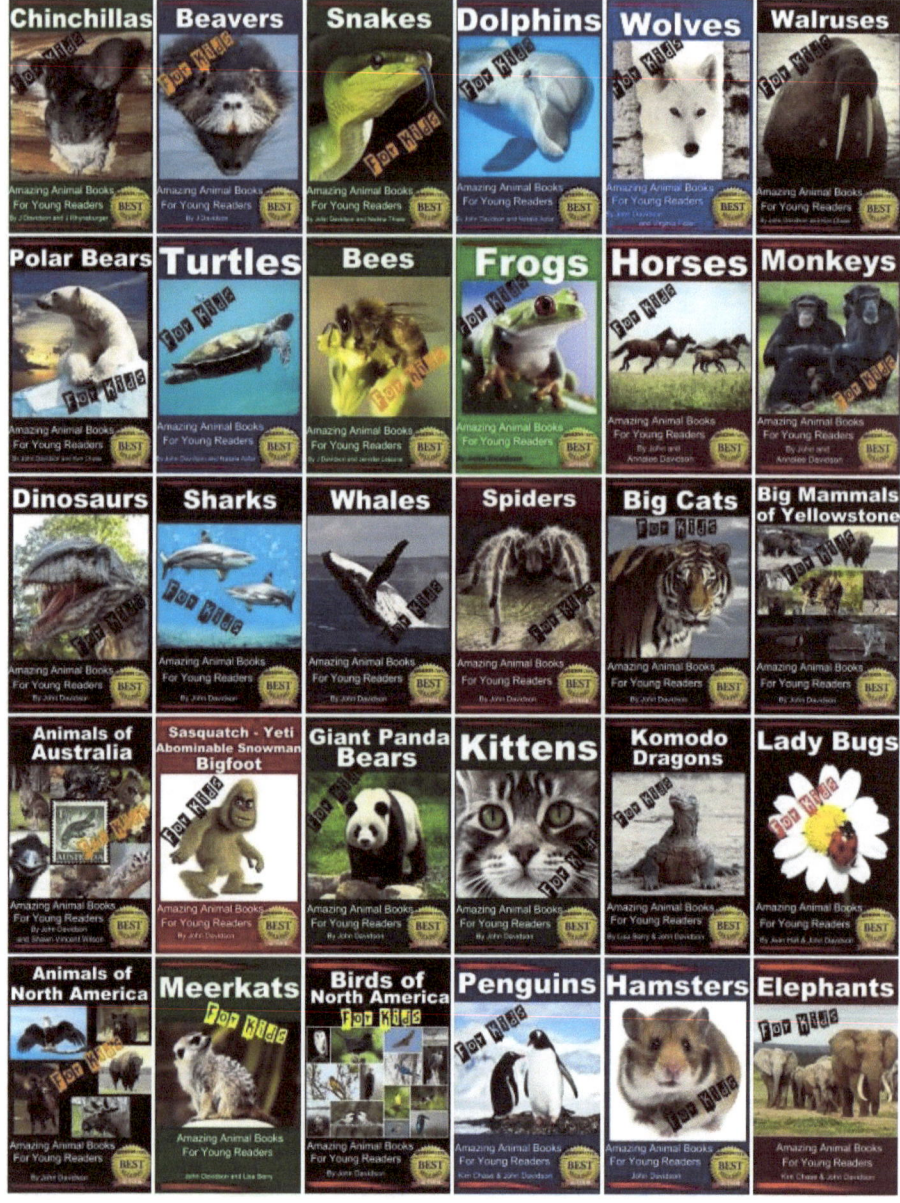

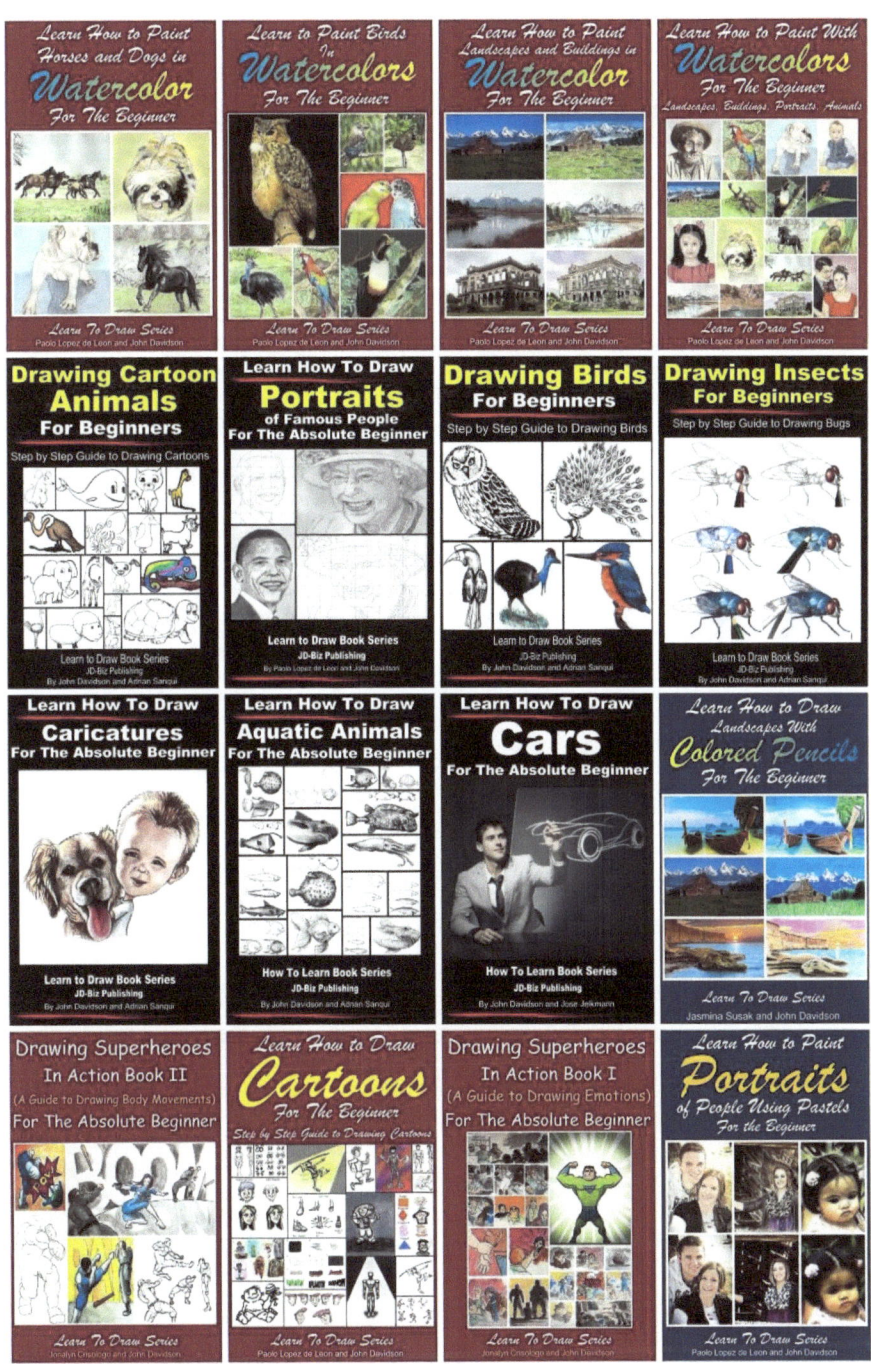

How to Build and Plan Books

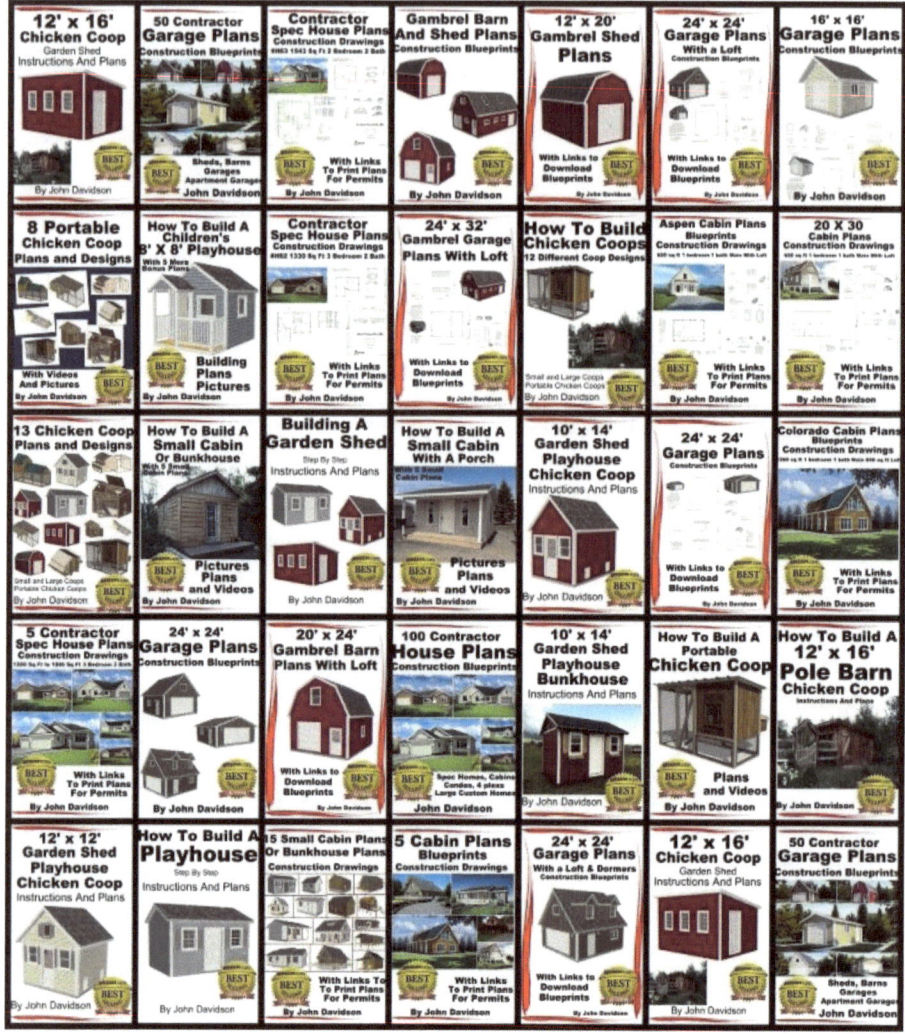

Entrepreneur Book Series

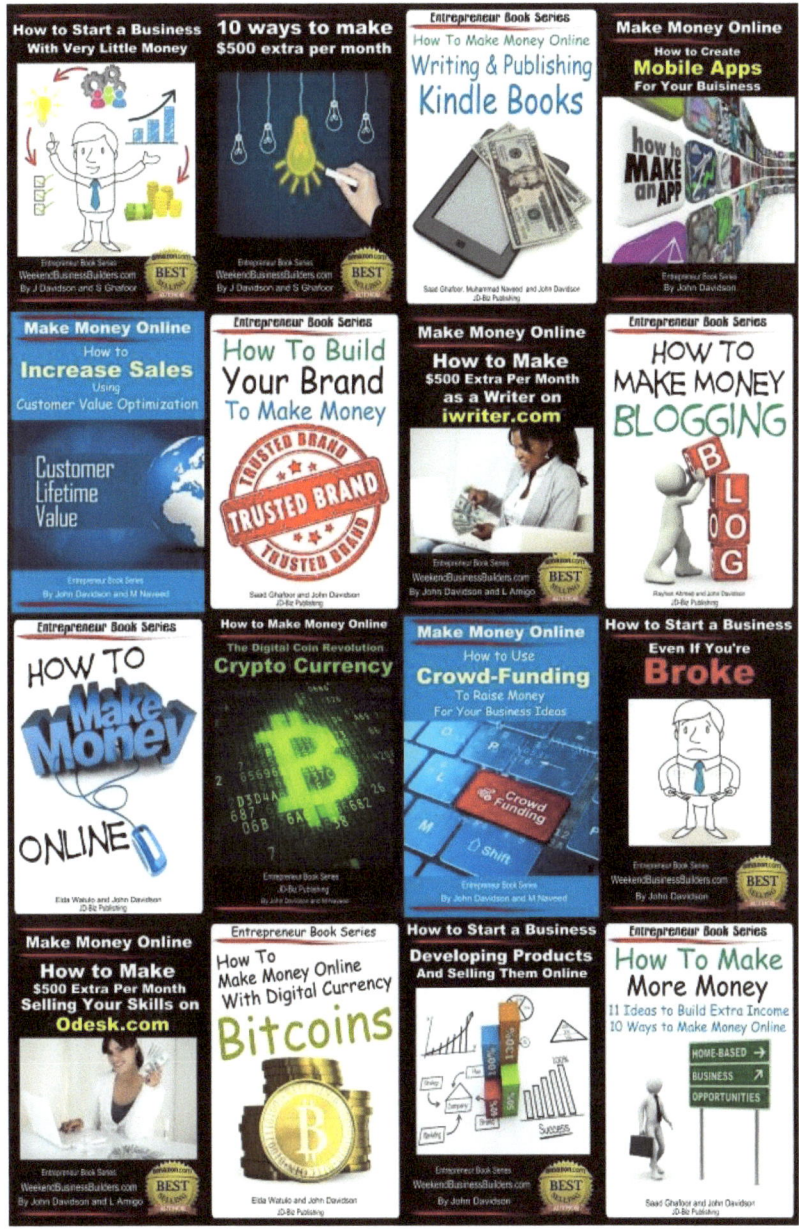

Our books are available at

1. Amazon.com

2. Barnes and Noble

3. Itunes

4. Kobo

5. Smashwords

6. Google Play Books

Download Free Books!

http://MendonCottageBooks.com

Publisher

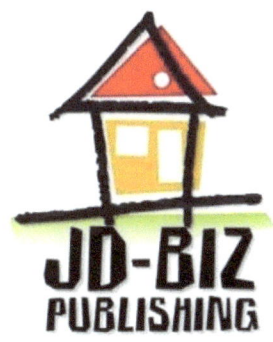

JD-Biz Corp

P O Box 374

Mendon, Utah 84325

http://www.jd-biz.com/

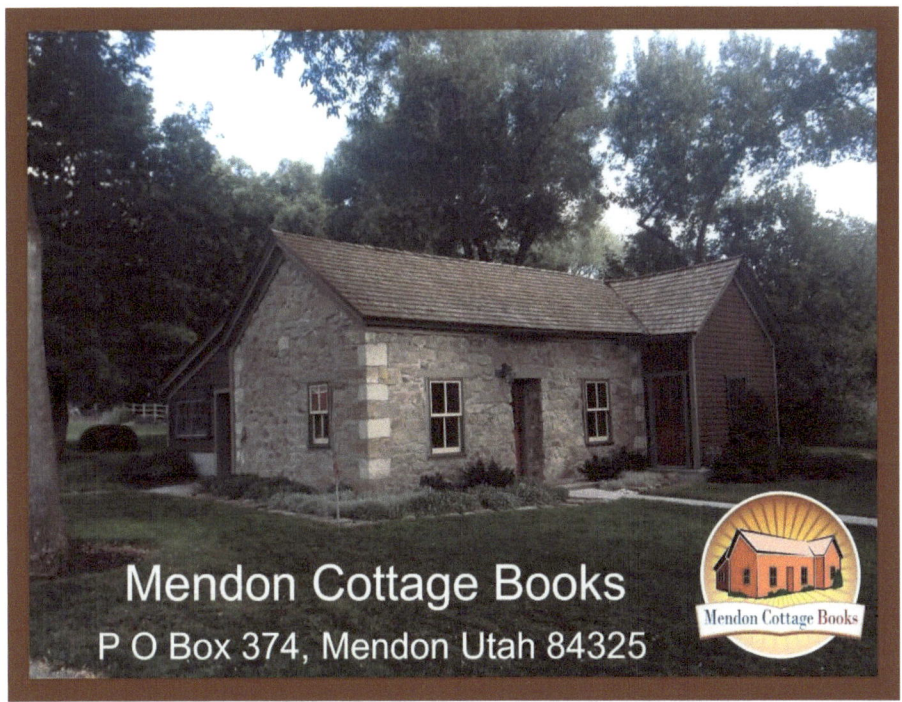

www.ingramcontent.com/pod-product-compliance
Lightning Source LLC
Chambersburg PA
CBHW050840290526
45792CB00001B/475